WHY VEGAN DIET

Amin Heidari

DEDICATION

THIS BOOK IS DEDICATED TO YOU—BOLD SOULS WHO'VE OPTED TO NOURISH YOURSELVES WITH THE EXTRAORDINARY POTENCY OF PLANTS. YOUR DEDICATION TO A VEGAN LIFESTYLE NOT ONLY SHOWCASES YOUR CARE FOR ANIMALS AND THE EARTH BUT ALSO SHOWCASES THE PROFOUND INFLUENCE THAT MINDFUL DIETARY CHOICES CAN WIELD OVER OUR OWN WELL-BEING.

WITHIN THESE PAGES, WE HONOR THE WONDERS OF VEGANISM AND ITS UNDENIABLE ADVANTAGES FOR OUR PHYSICAL HEALTH. FROM THE DYNAMIC VITALITY SURGING THROUGH YOUR VEINS TO THE RADIANT LUMINOSITY GRACING YOUR SKIN, YOUR RESOLVE TO PRIORITIZE PLANT-BASED NOURISHMENT STANDS AS A TESTAMENT TO THE REMARKABLE METAMORPHOSIS POSSIBLE WHEN OUR DIETS HARMONIZE WITH THE WISDOM OF NATURE.

CONTENTS

ACKNOWLEDGMENTS

Being vegan is a choice of reality.
Not a choice of option.

GAINING INSIGHT INTO VEGANISM

Veganism, a luminous journey that unfurls beyond the boundaries of being merely a philosophy or lifestyle, beckons us to venture into a realm of profound comprehension, igniting our awareness of the intricate threads that weave us into the rich tapestry of the world. This transformative odyssey stretches far beyond the realms of mere dietary preferences, guiding us toward a life steeped in compassion, mindfulness, and a heightened connection to the intricate fabric of existence. As we embark on this enlightening expedition of gaining insight into veganism, we take our first steps on a path that interweaves multiple dimensions of our lives – embracing not only the nourishment of our bodies and ethical considerations but delving into the realms of nutrition, gastronomy, and the intricate web of the environment.

At the core of veganism resides an unwavering stance against cruelty and exploitation, standing as a testament to the deeply rooted belief that every sentient being, regardless of its form, merits reverence and empathy. By embracing the abundance of plant-based foods, we proclaim our allegiance to a worldview that transcends individual preferences and sets a tone for a collective recognition of the sanctity of all life forms. This compels us to peer beyond our plates, delving into the intricate interconnectedness of our choices and fostering an understanding that our dietary decisions resonate far beyond our immediate nourishment, echoing through the complex ecosystems of our planet and influencing the delicate balance of life that sustains us all.

This journey of comprehending veganism extends far beyond a mere intellectual exercise; it becomes a dynamic voyage of self-discovery and perpetual learning. It urges us to navigate the labyrinthine nuances of plant-based diets, to unearth the diverse sources that offer essential nutrients, and to challenge the misconception that animal products are the exclusive bearers of vitality. This expedition empowers us to curate meals that not only nurture our bodies but also nourish our souls and foster harmony with the natural world, nurturing a union of health and sustainability that resonates through our daily actions and choices.

Veganism invites us to awaken the artist within, to paint on the canvas of our kitchens with a vibrant and diverse palette of plant-based ingredients. The spectrum of flavors, textures, and culinary possibilities unfurls like a symphony of tastes, allowing us to craft culinary creations that rival even the most cherished traditional cuisines. This exploration transcends the realm of taste, encapsulating the essence of innovation and creation, igniting a passion for culinary expression that resonates through each delicious bite and celebrates the symphony of flavors that nature generously provides.

Yet, veganism's canvas is expansive, reaching beyond the individual plate to encompass the vast terrain of our planet's well-being. It casts a spotlight on the ecological footprint of animal agriculture – a resource-intensive practice that spans land use, water consumption, and greenhouse gas emissions. The adoption of a plant-based approach paints a brighter future, a world where our choices resonate with sustainability, creating a legacy that future generations will cherish and fostering a harmonious coexistence between humanity and the environment that nurtures and sustains us.

As we journey through life as conscious vegans, we learn the art of harmonizing our choices with social situations and engaging with the wider community. Armed with insight into veganism, we navigate social interactions with grace, articulate our choices with respect, and pave the way for understanding and acceptance among friends, family, and society. This journey empowers us to dine out with confidence, to seek vegan-friendly options, and to be catalysts for change through our actions and dialogues, sowing the seeds of transformation through our heartfelt conversations that ripple through the fabric of our relationships and societal norms.

The essence of gaining insight into veganism extends beyond a finite horizon; it is a continuous expedition of personal growth and metamorphosis. It stands as a commitment to fuse our values with our everyday decisions, heralding a world defined by compassion, sustainability, and justice. Through this transformative journey, we nourish not only our bodies but also our minds and spirits, cultivating a profound realization of the intricate interconnectedness that binds all life forms, unveiling the vibrant mosaic of existence that extends beyond our personal horizons. It's a melody that resonates through time, inviting us to be stewards of a future that reflects the harmonious unity of all beings and celebrates the beauty of a world embraced by compassion and conscious living, a world where our actions ripple with meaning, and our choices resonate as notes in the symphony of life that we collectively compose and conduct.

THE NUTRIENT BASIS OF A PLANT-BASED DIET

plant-based diet, intricately woven into the fabric of nature's offerings, unfolds as a harmonious symphony of nourishment and well-being. Beyond a simple dietary preference, it evolves into a holistic lifestyle that reveres the intricate interplay of nutrients as the essence of vitality. The nutrient basis of a plant-based diet is a resounding affirmation of the extraordinary potential that plant-derived foods possess to provide a comprehensive spectrum of essential elements critical for our optimal health and flourishing.

At the heart of this nutrient-rich approach lies a vivid tapestry of vital components, each contributing harmoniously to support every facet of our well-being. Plant-based foods, resplendent in their diverse colors, textures, and flavors, deliver a symphony of nutrients that collaborate synergistically to maintain our physiological equilibrium. Far from isolated units, these nutrients dance together to foster vibrant health, resilience, and longevity.

Central to the nutrient foundation of a plant-based diet are the vitamins and minerals, the fundamental micronutrients that fuel our cells, optimize metabolic processes, and finely orchestrate the functioning of our organs. From the immune-boosting embrace of vitamin C found in vibrant citrus fruits to the bone-nurturing qualities of calcium inherent in dark leafy greens, plant-based sources present a treasure trove of nutrients that fortify our bodies from the inside out.

Equally pivotal are the complex carbohydrates that characterize a substantial portion of plant-based foods. These carbohydrates serve as the life force of sustained energy, propelling our daily activities and ensuring a steady cognitive rhythm. The remarkable presence of dietary fiber, intrinsic to plant-based sources, functions as a natural cleanser for our digestive system, promoting gut health, aiding in the delicate balance of blood sugar levels, and bestowing a sense of satiety that empowers effective weight management.

The grandeur of the nutrient basis extends to the realm of proteins, the elemental building blocks of life. Thriving within plant-based sources such as legumes, grains, nuts, and seeds, these proteins provide not only a plentiful supply but also an exquisite diversity of amino acids, vital for tissue repair, immune resilience, and the comprehensive growth and regeneration of the body.

Among the pantheon of essential nutrients, fatty acids claim their significance within the nutrient foundation of a plant-based diet. Omega-3 fatty acids, renowned for their cardiovascular and neurocognitive advantages, are readily accessible through plant sources like flaxseeds, chia seeds, and walnuts. These fatty acids contribute to the vitality of our cardiovascular system, foster cognitive acuity, and play a pivotal role in modulating the body's inflammatory responses.

Venturing deeper into the spectrum, plant-based diets offer a profusion of antioxidants, powerful compounds found in the kaleidoscope of colorful fruits and vegetables. These guardians of cellular well-being combat the rigors of oxidative stress and inflammation, serving as sentinels against chronic ailments and fortifying the body's innate defense mechanisms.

Furthermore, the nutrient basis of a plant-based diet embraces an array of phytonutrients, bioactive compounds that bestow a plethora of health advantages. From anti-inflammatory properties to immune fortification, these plant-derived marvels exemplify the intricate interplay between diet and well-being, underscoring the substantial impact of our dietary choices on our overall health and longevity.

To embrace the nutrient foundation of a plant-based diet is to embark on a journey of empowerment and enlightenment. It involves a conscious decision to nourish our bodies with the bounty that nature provides, recognizing that the intricate interplay of these nutrients fosters a state of optimal health and balance. Through the exploration of a diverse array of plant-based foods, we embark on a culinary voyage that not only delights our palates but also bolsters our overall vitality.

In a world brimming with culinary wonders, the nutrient basis of a plant-based diet unveils a vibrant tapestry of nutrients that stand as a testament to the power of conscious dietary choices. It reinforces the profound connection between our plates and our health, emphasizing the importance of aligning our diets with the rhythms of nature in our pursuit of well-being. As we navigate this transformative path, we come to understand that the earth's bounty is a true ally in nurturing our bodies, empowering us to lead lives that resonate with balance, vitality, and enduring health, echoing the symphony of nature's wisdom within ourselves.

Strategizing Meals and Ready-To-Eat Preparations

Within the realm of embracing a plant-based lifestyle, the art of orchestrating meals and welcoming the practicality of ready-to-eat preparations emerges as a potent duo. This dynamic approach not only ensures a well-rounded and nourishing diet but also equips us to seamlessly navigate our bustling lives with grace and efficiency.

The Choreography of Meal Planning:

Meal planning in the context of a plant-based journey extends beyond logistics; it evolves into a symphony of flavors, nutrients, and ingenuity. This process involves envisaging a palette of balanced meals, rich in colors, textures, and vital elements. By thoughtfully integrating an array of fruits, vegetables, whole grains, legumes, nuts, and seeds, we embark on a culinary expedition that not only nurtures our bodies but also tantalizes our taste buds.

The essence of meal planning lies in celebrating diversity. By artfully combining ingredients, we not only embrace a range of nutrients but also stave off monotony, ensuring that our culinary experience remains engaging and fulfilling. Seasonal produce breathes life into our dishes, connecting us with the rhythms of nature and infusing our meals with an invigorating essence.

A well-designed plant-based meal is a tapestry that interweaves crucial macronutrients – carbohydrates, proteins, and wholesome fats – in a harmonious dance. Hearty whole grains like quinoa and brown rice, in partnership with legumes such as lentils and chickpeas, constitute the bedrock of sustenance. Meanwhile, the richness of nuts, seeds, and avocados imparts a tapestry of healthy fats. When paired with an array of vibrant vegetables, these components converge to craft a culinary masterpiece that not only fuels our bodies but also delights our senses.

Embracing the Ease of Ready-to-Eat Preparations:

In the whirlwind of modern life, the concept of ready-to-eat preparations emerges as a beacon of practicality. This entails prepping components of our meals in advance, ensuring that nourishing choices are readily accessible, even in the face of time constraints. Whether it involves dicing vegetables, pre-cooking grains, or assembling salads, these small yet strategic efforts can dramatically enhance our ability to maintain a seamless plant-based lifestyle.

Ready-to-eat preparations empower us to circumvent the allure of less nutritious options when confronted with time limitations. Whether it's a premade salad, a batch of cooked quinoa, or an assortment of sliced fruits, these choices not only offer a swift and nourishing solution but also shield us from impulsive selections that might deviate from our dietary aspirations.

Navigating the Plant-Based Pantry:

A well-organized pantry forms the bedrock of effective meal planning and ready-to-eat readiness. By stocking up on vital plant-based essentials like grains, legumes, nuts, seeds, and an assortment of spices, we lay the groundwork for a versatile culinary journey. Staples like canned beans, frozen vegetables, and plant-based milk serve as invaluable resources for constructing well-balanced meals, especially during busier times.

Igniting Creativity:

Strategizing meals and embracing the convenience of ready-to-eat solutions invites our innate creativity to flourish. Experimenting with diverse flavors, textures, and cooking methods transforms meal preparation into a delightful voyage of culinary discovery. By embracing new recipes and diverse culinary traditions, we cultivate a sense of wonder that infuses each mealtime with joy and anticipation.

In summation, the synergy between crafting meal strategies and embracing ready-to-eat convenience forms a robust foundation for a thriving plant-based lifestyle. This approach empowers us to savor an array of nutrients, uphold a well-rounded diet, and navigate our daily routines with seamless efficiency. Beyond mere sustenance, these practices become gateways to a life that celebrates health, vibrancy, and the pleasure of relishing the richness that plant-based cuisine offers.

HARMONY WITH THE PLANET AND ETHICAL CONSIDERATIONS

The journey towards a plant-based lifestyle extends far beyond personal health; it's a transformative voyage that intertwines with the very fabric of our planet and resonates with ethical considerations that touch the hearts of all living beings. This conscious choice not only nurtures our own well-being but also becomes a resounding testament to our commitment to fostering harmony, sustainability, and compassion.

Harmonizing with the Planet:

At the heart of embracing a plant-based lifestyle lies a harmonious dance with the Earth's intricate ecosystems. Animal agriculture, with its vast land requirements, substantial water consumption, and significant greenhouse gas emissions, casts a considerable environmental shadow. Opting for a plant-based approach signifies an acknowledgment of our responsibility towards reducing our impact on the planet's finite resources. Plant cultivation generally demands less land and water, while emitting fewer greenhouse gases compared to the demands of animal farming. By aligning our dietary choices with the well-being of the planet, we actively contribute to the preservation of biodiversity, the protection of fragile habitats, and the sustenance of ecosystems that are the bedrock of our existence.

Moreover, a plant-based diet embodies a circular model of nourishment. Choosing plants over animal products redirects resources away from animal agriculture, channeling them towards feeding more individuals directly. This shift fosters efficiency, reduces wastage, and supports a food system that not only sustains us but also respects the delicate balance of the natural world.

Nurturing Ethical Considerations:

Ethics stands as a foundational pillar of the plant-based philosophy, reflecting a profound commitment to empathy and compassion for every sentient being. Embracing a plant-based lifestyle stems from an awareness that animals raised for food possess emotions, experience pain, and hold inherent value. Opting for nourishment derived from plants signifies a deliberate choice to minimize the exploitation and suffering of fellow beings.

By consciously abstaining from animal products, we detach our support from industries that often perpetuate practices inconsistent with our values of compassion. The intensive confinement systems and profit-driven practices of animal farming are often at odds with the principles of empathy and respect for life.

The ethical dimension of a plant-based lifestyle transcends individual dietary choices; it extends into the realm of advocacy and education. Our choices are a testament to our commitment to positive change, inspiring others to reevaluate their connections to animals and the environment. Our actions reverberate through our communities, igniting conversations, spreading awareness, and sparking discussions about animal welfare and planetary stewardship.

In essence, the harmonious fusion of a plant-based lifestyle, environmental consciousness, and ethical considerations shapes a paradigm that surpasses personal well-being. It encapsulates a holistic approach to thriving that recognizes the interconnectedness of all life forms and the delicate balance of our planet's ecosystems. By embracing this ethos, we not only nourish our bodies but also cultivate a world rooted in compassion, sustainability, and a profound understanding of our role within the magnificent tapestry of life. In our quest for well-being, we stand as stewards of a future where harmony and ethical consciousness flourish, enriching both our lives and the world we call home.

Navigating Supplements and Enriched Nourishment

The Complex Terrain of Supplements:

Supplements, evolving in response to the contemporary pursuit of comprehensive well-being, stand as a testament to humanity's quest for optimized vitality. They materialize as answers to bridge the gaps that may exist within our nutritional intake, offering specialized support to target specific health nuances. Within this expansive realm, a tapestry of possibilities is woven, embracing an assortment of vitamins, minerals, herbal extracts, amino acids, and an array of other bioactive compounds. This captivating diversity ensures that the spectrum of preferences and necessities is not only acknowledged but also catered to, manifested in an array of forms ranging from the convenience of pills and capsules to the novelty of powders and gummies.

However, amidst this abundance, a discerning eye becomes indispensable. The landscape reveals a dual nature: some supplements, buoyed by the weight of empirical validation, stand as veritable allies in the journey toward wellness. Others, however, dance on the periphery, cloaked in the shimmering attire of marketing claims. The ability to navigate this labyrinthine space, distinguishing between evidence-based supplements and the ephemeral allure of trends, has morphed into an essential aptitude in an era awash with information. As seekers of holistic health, we are entrusted with the responsibility of peeling away the layers, unveiling the gems of science from the veneer of marketing, as we embark on the path to a more informed and nourished existence.

Balancing Benefits and Risks:

The potential benefits of supplements, when embraced with careful consideration, unfold as a realm of undeniable promise. They offer a lifeline, delivering essential nutrients that might otherwise remain elusive due to dietary restrictions, lifestyle choices, or underlying medical circumstances. Consider individuals committed to rigorous dietary regimens; their pursuit of well-being may necessitate supplementation to fortify against potential deficiencies. Likewise, in the dynamic arena of physical performance, athletes deftly employ the potential of protein and amino acid supplements, harnessing these tools to amplify recovery efforts and propel themselves toward the zenith of their capabilities.

Yet, on this journey towards vitality, the road is not without its cautionary markers. As we blend supplements into our wellness mosaic, an acute awareness of potential pitfalls is imperative. The act of combining various supplements without a thorough assessment of their potential interactions can unwittingly sow the seeds for adverse outcomes. The notion of "more is better" holds no truer than in the case of vitamins or minerals—a practice known as mega-dosing. This path, while trodden with the best of intentions, can lead to a delicate balance disrupted, paving the way for toxicity and imbalances that imperil well-being.

In the light of these intricacies, a partnership with healthcare professionals assumes its significance. They emerge as skilled navigators, steering the ship of supplementation through treacherous waters. Their expert guidance ensures that the supplementation chosen is tailored to individual needs and aspirations. Moreover, these professionals stand as vigilant sentinels, safeguarding against disharmony with medications and pre-existing health conditions.

In summation, the realm of supplements stands as a double-edged sword, one that can be a potent ally when wielded judiciously or a potential threat when wielded recklessly. With each step taken towards a healthier self, the counsel of healthcare professionals and the wisdom to navigate the seas of supplementation can elevate this journey from a mere quest for wellness to a harmonious symphony of nourishment and vitality.

The Significance of Enriched Nourishment:
Within the intricate tapestry of health and nutrition, the concept of enriched nourishment emerges as a guiding light, illuminating the path toward collective well-being. Fortified foods, standing at the intersection of community needs and industry innovation, embody a

solution to the pressing challenge of nutritional deficits. These foods, once simple staples like cereals, dairy products, and plant-based alternatives, now undergo a metamorphosis, emerging imbued with an arsenal of essential nutrients that act as vital building blocks for optimal health. Whether it's the sunlit embrace of vitamin D or the steadfast strength of iron, these nutrients infuse these everyday foods with newfound potential.

This strategic approach serves as a counterbalance to the complex factors that contribute to nutritional inadequacies. Dietary choices, influenced by diverse cultural preferences and individual constraints, often fall short of providing the full spectrum of nutrients needed for vibrant health. Socioeconomic circumstances can also limit access to a diverse range of nutrient-rich foods, thereby exacerbating the challenge. In this landscape, fortified foods bridge the gap, ensuring that regardless of dietary choices or economic limitations, essential nutrients are readily available to all.

Embracing enriched nourishment marks a collective commitment to empowering individuals with the tools they need to thrive. It encapsulates a synergy between nutritional science, culinary creativity, and a shared understanding that health is not a privilege but a fundamental right. As communities unite around this concept, fortified foods emerge not just as products but as agents of positive change, nourishing not only bodies but also the potential for a brighter, healthier future for all.

ENGAGING IN SOCIAL SETTINGS AND EATING OUT

The Essence of Dining Together:

Beyond being a mere source of sustenance, sharing a meal transcends into a captivating symphony, where flavors harmonize with conversations, laughter, and the art of forging connections. The spectrum of dining experiences stretches from the warmth of intimate family dinners to the opulence of celebratory feasts, and from the coziness of romantic dates to the purposeful gatherings of professional luncheons. Within this realm of shared sustenance, every morsel and every moment intertwine, weaving threads of strength into the tapestry of relationships. It's in these shared meals that camaraderie is nurtured, and cherished memories are crafted, indelibly etching themselves into the chapters of our lives.

This communal experience of breaking bread extends its tendrils beyond the table, reaching deep into the heart of communities. Just as the pieces of a puzzle come together to form a beautiful picture, the act of dining together solidifies bonds between individuals, bridging gaps and fostering a profound sense of belonging. It's a unifying ritual, irrespective of backgrounds, cultures, or beliefs. In these moments, barriers are softened, and the simple act of enjoying a meal becomes a universal language that speaks of our shared humanity.

The very essence of these shared meals is the embodiment of unity, a reminder that despite the hustle of life, the gathering around a table allows for genuine connections to flourish. As conversations flow, stories are exchanged, and laughter echoes, the richness of these experiences extends far beyond the culinary delights. They become a testament to our shared need for connection, reminding us that the simple act of dining together is a celebration of life's shared moments and an affirmation of the bonds that tie us all together.

Embarking on a Culinary Exploration:

Entering the realm of dining out is akin to embarking on a thrilling expedition through the world of flavors and gastronomy. As one crosses the threshold of restaurants, cafes, and eateries, a captivating tapestry of global cuisines unfurls, showcasing a diverse array of dishes that traverse cultures, flavors, and culinary techniques. This journey is a sensory adventure that engages taste buds, ignites curiosity, and stimulates the senses in delightful ways.

The odyssey commences with the tantalizing act of perusing menus, where each page presents a novel chapter in the culinary story. The artful descriptions and vibrant imagery of the dishes create a symphony of anticipation. With each selection, one makes a conscious choice, guided by personal preferences and adventurous spirit. The act of choosing becomes a moment of anticipation, as the forthcoming flavors and aromas are unveiled like precious gems in a treasure trove.

As the dishes are served, the experience transforms into a multisensory spectacle. The play of colors on the plate, the aromatic dance that wafts through the air, and the textures that greet the palate—all contribute to an orchestration of sensations. It's not just a meal; it's a journey of flavors, an exploration of culinary artistry, and an immersion into the culture from which each dish originates.

Beyond the indulgence lies the educational aspect of this journey. Each dish carries a history, a tradition, and a story that transcends its ingredients. Dining out offers an opportunity to learn about the rich tapestry of cuisines that populate our world. The flavors speak of the land, the techniques tell of culinary wisdom passed down through generations, and the fusion of ingredients is a testament to the cross-pollination of cultures.

Yet, the true magic of dining out lies in its capacity to transcend comfort zones. It's an invitation to step beyond the familiar and embrace the uncharted territories of taste. Just as travel broadens the mind, venturing beyond culinary comfort zones broadens the palate. In this realm, even the most seasoned gastronomes find themselves surprised and delighted by new taste sensations.

Ultimately, stepping into the world of dining out is an adventure that enriches both the senses and the soul. It's an exploration that satiates curiosity, nurtures appreciation for the artistry of food, and brings the world's flavors to our doorstep. It's a reminder that the journey of food is an eternal one, a continuous exploration of flavors, cultures, and the sheer joy of indulgence.

Striking a Balance Amid Temptations:

However, while the world of dining out promises excitement, it also presents a set of nuanced challenges. The enchanting allure of indulging in delectable dishes, coupled with the generous portion sizes and the tantalizing allure of sumptuous ingredients, can inadvertently pave the way to overindulgence. The very factors that make dining out so enticing can become potential pitfalls, testing our self-discipline and ability to moderate our consumption.
Moreover, navigating the landscape of menus, though exciting, can also prove to be a delicate endeavor. The array of options, each brimming with its unique flavor profile and allure, beckons us to explore. Yet, aligning these choices with personal dietary preferences, health goals, or nutritional considerations requires a discerning eye. It's a balancing act that demands a thoughtful examination of ingredients, preparation methods, and portion sizes.

In this intricate web of culinary delights, the art of balance emerges as a key protagonist. The quest to satisfy our taste buds and nourish our bodies converges into a delicate dance. The desire to savor every bite must be tempered with the intention to make choices that align with our broader well-being objectives. The pursuit of enjoyment must harmonize with the awareness of our nutritional needs. This fusion of pleasure and prudence creates a symphony of mindful choices that can define the outcome of our dining experiences.

As we navigate these culinary landscapes, embracing the pleasures of dining out while upholding our personal health aspirations, our choices are a testament to our commitment to holistic well-being. Each menu selection, each consideration of portion size, and every moment of choosing moderation over excess reflects our dedication to striking a harmonious equilibrium. And in this delicate art of balancing desire with intention, we find empowerment—a reminder that we have the agency to navigate the world of dining out with both enjoyment and mindful control.

OPTIMAL FITNESS AND THE VEGAN LIFESTYLE

A Plant-Powered Foundation:

Wholeheartedly adopting the vegan lifestyle signifies a deliberate decision to remove animal products from one's dietary choices. At the core of this approach lies plant-based eating, a philosophy that places an emphasis on deriving nourishment from nature's offerings: fruits, vegetables, grains, legumes, nuts, and seeds. These ingredients, brimming with a vibrant assortment of vitamins, minerals, antioxidants, and dietary fiber, become the bedrock of sustenance, offering a complete and diverse array of nutrients without reliance on sources derived from animals.

The beauty of plant-based eating is its inherent harmony with both individual aspirations and broader global responsibilities. This very foundation resonates profoundly with those who are not only dedicated to maximizing their fitness potential but also committed to upholding their ethical convictions and acknowledging the environmental impact of their dietary choices.

By adopting a vegan lifestyle, individuals are choosing more than just sustenance; they are embracing a lifestyle that aligns their plate with their values. The decision to omit animal products is not solely about what's being consumed; it becomes a statement of compassion toward animals, acknowledging their intrinsic worth and avoiding their exploitation. Moreover, it becomes an expression of environmental consciousness, acknowledging the significant reduction in resource consumption, greenhouse gas emissions, and land use associated with plant-based diets.

For those striving for optimal fitness, this ethical and ecological alignment takes on a unique significance. The very choices made to fuel their bodies are intertwined with a commitment to the greater good. The plant-based foundation, rich in essential nutrients, lays the groundwork for muscle development, energy sustainability, and overall well-being, all while contributing to the planet's well-being.

This intersection of principles and practicality underscores that adopting the vegan lifestyle isn't just about swapping ingredients—it's about reshaping one's relationship with food, ethics, and the environment. As each plate of plant-based goodness is savored, it becomes a reflection of a conscious and compassionate approach to living. It's an embodiment of the belief that optimizing one's own well-being can harmoniously coexist with fostering a healthier planet for all beings to thrive.

Nutritional Considerations:

The harmonious relationship between achieving optimal fitness and embracing the vegan lifestyle is intricately woven through the art of nutrient curation. This meticulous process involves not only selecting the right foods but also understanding how they synergize to support physical well-being. At the heart of this fusion lies an array of nutrients that collectively contribute to vitality and strength.

Protein, often hailed as a cornerstone in the fitness journey, effortlessly finds its place within the plant-based realm. A variety of sources, including legumes, tofu, tempeh, quinoa, and nuts, offer ample protein to facilitate muscle repair and growth. This protein diversity ensures that all essential amino acids are accounted for, allowing the body to effectively utilize these building blocks for various physiological processes.

Carbohydrates, often regarded as the body's primary source of energy, play a crucial role in fueling workouts and facilitating post-exercise recovery. Whole grains, rich in complex carbohydrates, provide sustained energy release, enabling individuals to engage in workouts with vigor and endure longer durations of physical activity. These carbohydrates also aid in replenishing glycogen stores, contributing to quicker recovery and readiness for subsequent sessions.

Healthy fats, deriving their goodness from sources like avocados, nuts, and seeds, play a dual role in the vegan fitness equation. They contribute to satiety, helping individuals manage hunger and maintain stable energy levels throughout the day. Beyond that, these fats supply essential fatty acids that support cell health, hormone production, and cognitive function.

The crux of this nutritional symphony lies in maintaining a delicate balance and variety of nutrients. The vegan diet's richness in plant-derived antioxidants, vitamins, and minerals further bolsters overall health, reducing the oxidative stress that can accompany intense physical training. By thoughtfully curating meals that encompass a spectrum of colors and nutrients, individuals can harness the power of plant-based foods to fortify their bodies from the inside out.

In the realm of veganism and fitness, education becomes a powerful tool. Understanding the nutrients that one's body requires, and how to obtain them from plant sources, paves the way for success. Mindful meal planning ensures that nutrient needs are met, ultimately laying the groundwork for muscle development, energy sustainability, and holistic vitality.

Ultimately, this symbiosis is a testament to the potential of the vegan lifestyle to complement and enhance the pursuit of optimal fitness. It's a synergy that underscores the versatility of plant-based foods and the inherent capacity of the body to thrive on this compassionate and nourishing path.

Ethical Wellness and Environmental Stewardship:

Adopting the vegan lifestyle transcends the realm of mere dietary choices; it's a profound ethical pledge that embraces compassion for sentient beings and a deliberate stride towards preserving the planet's delicate balance. This commitment reverberates far beyond personal health considerations, resonating deeply with the interconnectedness of all life forms and the imperative of environmental stewardship. For a growing number of individuals, weaving the tapestry of fitness aspirations with the threads of vegan values creates a powerful synergy that extends beyond the realm of physical well-being.

The decision to intertwine fitness goals with veganism arises from a wellspring of compassion. It's a stance that recognizes the inherent worth of every creature, extending kindness not just to humanity but to all sentient beings. This ethical commitment reverberates throughout one's choices, serving as a reminder that every meal is an opportunity to uphold these values and make a difference, not just for personal transformation but for the greater good.

Environmental sustainability emerges as another cornerstone in this harmonious convergence. By choosing plant-based nourishment over animal-derived products, individuals are taking a conscious step towards reducing their ecological footprint. The process of animal agriculture, from land use and water consumption to greenhouse gas emissions, places an immense strain on the planet's resources. By opting for plant-based alternatives, individuals align their choices with a more sustainable future, contributing to the preservation of natural ecosystems and minimizing the negative impact on the environment.

This holistic approach, where individual health pursuits become intertwined with global consciousness, nurtures a profound sense of purpose. It's a realization that the journey towards personal well-being is inseparably linked to the well-being of the planet and its inhabitants. This interconnection becomes a wellspring of motivation, infusing each workout, each meal, and each lifestyle choice with a deeper sense of meaning.

Ultimately, the marriage of fitness goals and the vegan lifestyle encapsulates a philosophy that's greater than the sum of its parts. It's a path that emanates from a heart that beats in rhythm with compassion, that seeks harmony with the natural world, and that acknowledges the interdependence of all life forms. This alignment of personal transformation and global responsibility forms a tapestry that's woven with threads of purpose, resilience, and a commitment to leaving a positive imprint on the planet.

The Role of Mindfulness:

Embracing optimal fitness while adhering to a vegan lifestyle necessitates a heightened level of mindfulness that transcends the boundaries of the plate. It's not solely about what one consumes but also about recognizing how those choices align with broader ethical, environmental, and health values. This practice of mindful eating becomes a powerful conduit that connects physical nourishment with a profound awareness of the consequences of our dietary decisions.

Mindful eating within the vegan framework is more than just a trend; it's a way of cultivating a deep connection with the food we consume. It's an act of reverence for the Earth's resources and the lives that are affected by our choices. With each bite, there's an opportunity to express gratitude for the sustenance that the Earth provides while being conscious of the impact of our dietary preferences on the planet's delicate ecosystems.

This level of mindfulness extends beyond the mere act of eating; it permeates every facet of the vegan fitness journey. From the selection of ingredients to the preparation of meals, there's a deliberate intent to tread lightly on the Earth and honor all living beings. It's a reminder that every meal is a chance to make a statement, not only about our personal health but also about our commitment to global well-being.

In the realm of protein, often a focal point in fitness pursuits, this mindfulness manifests in the careful selection of plant-based sources. The awareness of complementary amino acids becomes paramount, ensuring that the protein sources chosen create a complete profile that supports muscle development, recovery, and overall well-being. This attentiveness reflects a dedication to understanding the intricacies of nutrition within the vegan paradigm and aligning these choices with fitness goals.

The amalgamation of optimal fitness, mindfulness, and the vegan lifestyle isn't just a lifestyle choice; it's a conscious evolution of one's relationship with food, values, and the planet. It's an intricate dance that underscores the potential of harnessing the power of plant-based nutrition not only for personal vitality but also as a means to contribute to a healthier world. It's a realization that the act of nourishing our bodies is intrinsically tied to nourishing the world around us—a testament to the harmonious synergy between individual well-being and global interconnectedness.

Embracing the Journey:

In the intricate tapestry woven by the merging pillars of optimal fitness and the vegan lifestyle, a powerful narrative of empowerment takes center stage. The journey becomes a living testament to the remarkable adaptability of the human body and spirit, showcasing that plant-based living is not only harmonious with vitality but also a gateway to unparalleled achievement in physical endeavors. From dedicated athletes to enthusiastic fitness aficionados, the intersection of a vegan lifestyle and optimal fitness becomes an inspiring invitation to transcend conventional boundaries and chart new territories of human potential.

At the heart of this journey lies a profound revelation: that our bodies are remarkably adaptable and responsive to the choices we make. The fusion of optimal fitness and the vegan lifestyle illuminates the innate capacity of the human body to thrive on a foundation of plant-powered sustenance. This realization dispels any lingering doubts and underscores that by adopting a vegan approach, we're providing our bodies with the nutrition it requires not just to survive, but to excel.

The narrative extends beyond individual achievements, embracing the broader impact of our choices. It's a celebration of how we, as individuals, can contribute to a healthier planet and a more compassionate society. The alignment of a vegan lifestyle with optimal fitness transcends personal gains, becoming a force that resonates through every stride taken and every rep completed, fostering a sense of purpose that extends beyond the gym walls.

The realm of athletics and fitness is no longer confined to conventional norms. Athletes and fitness enthusiasts alike are shattering stereotypes and redefining what it means to excel while embracing a plant-based lifestyle. They're showcasing that exceptional performance, muscular strength, and endurance are not exclusive to animal-derived nutrition. Instead, these achievements can be fueled by the vitality and resilience derived from whole plant foods.

This intersection is more than a juxtaposition; it's a harmonious integration that elevates both personal well-being and collective consciousness. It's an acknowledgment that choosing a vegan lifestyle isn't just about the pursuit of health, but an embodiment of a profound respect for the planet and all its inhabitants. It's an invitation to elevate our fitness aspirations to new heights while cultivating a profound reverence for the interconnectedness of all life.

Ultimately, the synergy between optimal fitness and the vegan lifestyle becomes an inspiring anthem of possibility. It's a declaration that the path to personal achievement need not be at odds with ethical convictions or environmental stewardship. It's a celebration of our capacity to adapt, thrive, and redefine our limits, all while honoring our bodies, our planet, and every living being that shares our journey.

THE END